Metab

Increase

Metabolism-Boosting Program for Speeding up Your Metabolism Through Exercise, Diet and Lifestyle So You Can Burn Fat, Build Muscle and Look and Feel Great

By Nathan Hollister

© **Copyright 2020 - All rights reserved.**

The content contained within this book may not be reproduced, duplicated or transmitted without direct written permission from the author or the publisher.

Under no circumstances will any blame or legal responsibility be held against the publisher or author for any damages, reparation, or monetary loss due to the information contained within this book. Either directly or indirectly.

Legal Notice:

This book is copyright protected. This book is only for personal use. You cannot amend, distribute, sell, use, quote or paraphrase any part, or the content within this book, without the consent of the author or publisher.

Disclaimer Notice:

Please note the information contained within this document is for educational and entertainment purposes only. All effort has been executed to present accurate, up to date and reliable, complete information. No warranties of any kind are declared or implied. Readers acknowledge that the author is not engaging in the rendering of legal, financial, medical or professional advice. The content within this book has been derived from various sources. Please consult a licensed professional before attempting any techniques outlined in this book.

By reading this document, the reader agrees that under no

circumstances is the author responsible for any losses, direct or indirect, which are incurred as a result of the use of information contained within this document, including, but not limited to, —errors, omissions, or inaccuracies.

Contents

INTRODUCTION 1

CHAPTER ONE: YOUR METABOLISM 2

    Metabolism Explained 2

    How Metabolism Functions 3

    Metabolism Types and Elements 3

    What Impacts Metabolism? 6

CHAPTER 2: WHY SHOULD YOU CARE ABOUT FIRING UP YOUR METABOLISM 9

CHAPTER 3: THE PROPER ATTITUDE 12

CHAPTER 4: IGNITING YOUR METABOLISM 15

    Metabolism Fuel # 1: Exercise Smart 16

        Strength and Resistance Training 17

        Interval Training 27

    Putting All of It Together 31

    Metabolism Fuel # 2: Eating Well 35

        Important Nutrients 36

        What to Stay Clear of 41

        Other Advised Foods 42

        Water is Key 43

        Timing is Important 44

        Sample Meal Plans 46

    Metabolism Fuel # 3: DE-STRESS 51

        Stress and Metabolism 52

        How to De-Stress 54

    Sleep is Essential 60

Conclusion 64

    Exercise Intelligently 65

    Eat Well. 65

    De-stress. 66

Thank you for buying this book and I hope that you will find it useful. If you will want to share your thoughts on this book, you can do so by leaving a review on the Amazon page, it helps me out a lot.

INTRODUCTION

If you know about about metabolism, odds are it was regarding weight loss. Metabolism is larger than losing weight, as you are going to find out eventually. It has to do with a much healthier, much greater you. If you wish to ignite your metabolism and you do not have a clue about how to do it, you arrived at the appropriate place. If you have attempted to accelerate your metabolism prior without noticeable effects, you have come to the appropriate place.

This guide is going to walk you through the essentials of metabolism and all that you have to do to accelerate your metabolism. Enjoy the journey!

CHAPTER ONE: YOUR METABOLISM

Metabolism Explained

Metabolism, in its most standard sense, is the body's transformation of the food calories into energy. It is a sequence of chain reactions which provide your body with the energy to do what it has to do to keep operating-- and subsequently, for you to stay alive. Without metabolism, you would not have the ability to think or move. Metabolism offers energy so that your body and organs can work properly.

To better comprehend the significance of metabolism, think about this: if your heart stops pounding, you pass away. Furthermore, if your metabolism ceases, you pass away-- since without metabolism, you are not going to have the energy to breathe or to ensure that your heart keeps on ponding!

How Metabolism Functions

Initially, let us begin with eating. As you swallow and chew your food, it heads to your digestive system. Digestive enzymes then break your food down -- carbs to glucose, protein into amino acids, and fats into fatty acids. After the nutrients are successfully broken down, they are taken in by the bloodstream and transported to the cells. Other enzymes, along with hormonal agents then function to either transform these nutrients into cells or tissue building blocks or discharge them as energy for the body's instantaneous utilization.

Metabolism Types and Elements

There are 2 fundamental metabolic procedures-- one is constructive, and is in charge of keeping and creating energy for the body. The other is destructive, although, in a good manner, as it breaks down nutrients to discharge energy. The constructive metabolic procedure is referred to as anabolism, while the destructive procedure is referred to as catabolism.

Anabolism stimulates the development of brand-new cells, the repair and maintenance of tissues, and the energy storage-- normally via body fat-- for future usage. Little nutrient molecules are transformed into bigger protein molecules, fat and carbs.

Catabolism, on the other hand, is in charge of offering the body the energy to utilize right away. Rather than building up, it breaks down the nutrient molecules to discharge energy.

These 2 procedures do not happen simultaneously, the body makes sure there is a balance between them. Catabolism, particularly, though certain people attribute this to total metabolism, has 3 elements:

1. Basal metabolism - Often referred to as resting metabolism, is the metabolism element behind maintaining you alive by guaranteeing typical body functions. Even if you were in bed the entire day, basal metabolism is still working.

Basal metabolism is metabolism's primary element, as two thirds of the calories from the food you consume are utilized for this. Individuals who wish to slim down typically go for a greater basal metabolic rate (BMR).

2. Physical motion - This could vary from a basic moving of your fingers to exhausting exercise. Typically, one quarter of the calories you take in go here.

3. Thermic impact of food - This points to the processing and digestion of the food you consume. Typically, ten percent of the calories you consume are burned through this. Therefore, taking all this into consideration, here is our formula for metabolism:

Calories From Food = Calories Used Up From Basal Metabolism (60-70%) + Calories Used Up By Physical Motion (25%) + Calories Used Up Digesting (10%).

What Impacts Metabolism?

Your metabolic rate, or how slowly or quickly your metabolism functions, is affected by a variety of elements:

1. Genes - Yes, the metabolic rate is additionally inherited. In some cases, this makes a whole world of distinction in between an individual who is able to eat practically anything and not acquire an ounce of fat and an individual who quickly balloons after indulging simply one time.

2. Age - The younger you are, the quicker your metabolism is. Metabolism decreases as you age. Female metabolic rate begins falling at 30; for guys, decrease begins later on at 40.

3. Gender - Guys have a quicker metabolic rate-- typically 10-15 percent quicker-- than women due to the fact that their bodies have a bigger muscle mass. Muscle plays a crucial role in quick metabolism, as it is going to be talked about in the chapter on working out.

4. Quantity of lean body mass - As pointed out above, more muscle = quicker metabolism.

5. Diet - Certain foods are going to assist you, some are just going to damage you. While timing is not all, when you consume additionally considerably impacts your metabolism. The distinction is gone over in part on eating properly.

6. Stress levels - Stress is inverse to metabolism. The more stress you go through, the lesser your metabolism. You are going to comprehend this better when we proceed to the section about stress.

7. Hormones - Particular hormones metabolize particular nutrients. How effectively the hormones function, then, impacts metabolism directly. To a particular level, diet plan and anxiety levels impact the hormones associated with metabolism, as you are going to learn later on. Hormonal imbalances or conditions can impact metabolism also.

Taking a look at all these aspects that affect metabolism, you now most likely have a rough idea of what you have to do to enhance your metabolism-- embrace the things you can not alter, and deal with those that you are able to!

However, prior to entering the comprehensive program for igniting your metabolism, initially, understand what's in it for you! And learn the type of determination you require to get the amount of metabolism you desire.

CHAPTER 2: WHY SHOULD YOU CARE ABOUT FIRING UP YOUR METABOLISM

It's not all about losing weight, though conversations on metabolism appear to focus nearly completely on this idea. Actually, even if you believe that your weight is completely fine, you have a great deal to get by boosting your metabolism. Here is a list of the benefits you can acquire by using the guidance in this guide:

1. Dropping weight. Let's begin with the most apparent advantage. By boosting your metabolism, especially your BMR, you are going to burn more calories simply by doing the activities you generally do. Even as you lie in bed staring at the ceiling, and even as you are asleep, your body is operating to burn the calories you take in. With a boost in metabolism, you could really shed a couple of pounds a week. Most importantly, the outcomes are long-lasting, unlike a quick-fix diet plan! Now, isn't that more gratifying-- and simpler-- than hopping on a fad diet?

2. Eating more without stressing over it - Because you burn calories quicker now, you could eat more without guilt. This does not suggest snacking on processed food or overindulging, however. In general, you could be less worried about the amount of food you consume.

3. Feeling more invigorated -Individuals with quicker metabolism report being more energetic. With a quicker metabolism, your body is operating effectively to release the energy you require to start.

4. Looking better - The skin of individuals with quick metabolism is more glowing and brighter. Their faces are pinkish, more alive with color. With a quicker metabolism, you are going to feel excellent while likewise looking great!

5. Better health in general - Your body works more effectively with a quicker metabolism. Food digestion, nutrients absorption, and blood flow are enhanced. And you won't require as much sleep as you did prior to feel revitalized the following day.

In sum, anticipate a quicker metabolism to make you feel and look more terrific.

CHAPTER 3: THE PROPER ATTITUDE

You are most likely questioning what all this has to do with attitude. Why not go straight to the guidance for boosting your metabolism?

The reason is that you have to be ready for what is ahead. Enhancing your metabolism is a big deal. It is no quick-fix diet plan where you just have to put in the effort for a couple of weeks-- and for certain diet plans, even for a couple of days.

Enhancing your metabolism has to do with altering your way of life and habits. Although you might select to begin with tiny changes, you are still going to be altering the lifestyle you have ended up being used to-- and it might feel unpleasant in the beginning. Enhancing your metabolism needs consistency and discipline in your actions. And considering that you are anticipating long-lasting outcomes, you are furthermore expected to make a long-term investment.

From here on, please take a look at the suggestions I am going to be giving you. You can not do just a few of them and still get the identical outcomes. The suggestions here abide by the gestalt principle, which says that the whole is greater than the sum of its parts. Believe that the elements of the program all function harmoniously to provide you with the preferred outcome.

So, now I wish for you to shut your eyes and picture yourself. Truly picture what you are going to be like after this program has actually begun to have an impact on you. How are you going to look? How are you going to feel?

Then, do the identical procedure for your expectations after 3 months, then 6 months-- and even a year, if you are able to. Observe the distinctions you feel and see.

It's a great idea to document your anticipated result. This is going to assist you in making it through the program, particularly when you are having a challenging time staying with the changes you formerly devoted yourself to.

Good job! You have started with the end in mind. This is going to considerably assist you along the road to your objective of igniting your metabolism.

CHAPTER 4: IGNITING YOUR METABOLISM

As I pointed out, please treat the guidance provided here as a whole program where you are going to have to use all the parts so as to increase your metabolism.

Initially, we are going to discuss exercise, as this is possibly the most important component of the program. Exercise done properly could significantly add to boosting your BMR. Here, you are going to find out how to exercise in a smart manner, and not constantly hard, as certain fitness programs may encourage. We are going to be discussing the significance of building muscle mass and using the perfect intensity to working out.

The second part has to do with eating properly, not about eating less, as certain weight reduction programs would encourage. You are going to discover that the outcomes you get are not going to just originate from the food you consume yet from when and how .

The last part has to do with dealing with stress. Some may see little value in this part. Understand, nevertheless, that stress is a strong and genuine obstacle to increasing your metabolism. Have this in mind as you go through this part.

Take some time to soak up every piece of guidance. You can begin using the suggestions here gradually, with the objective of placing everything together when your body has actually adjusted.

Metabolism Fuel # 1: Exercise Smart

Notice that I pointed out smart, not hard. Although certain exercises here might be high-intensity and might undoubtedly be tough for you, you don't have to work as hard and long as you might believe. The objective here is to ignite your metabolism with a workout program which takes the least amount of effort and time without compromising outcomes.

The two aspects of this workout program are resistance and strength training for growing lean muscle mass and interval training for accelerating the metabolism as a whole.

Strength and Resistance Training

The exercises in this training program are developed to develop resistance and strength, as the name recommends. Tension is administered to the muscles to attain this. The end outcome is boosted muscle mass in your body.

Building muscle is necessary as more muscle in your body implies more burned calories. Fitness specialist and trainer Robert Reames provides an ideal example by naming muscles fireplaces in the body which burn the fuel-- indicating calories. So the more fireplaces, the more fuel is burned. For each pound of muscle included, 50 more calories are burned each day.

Ladies don't need to stress over gaining big, unattractive muscles. Their bodies are not the same as male bodies. Female muscles are just going to include definition, and actually, make them look hotter.

While building muscles is generally tide to weightlifting, this is not constantly the instance. There are, in fact, numerous exercises which do not involve weights whatsoever. If you are on a tight budget plan, you could actually do exercises without any weights whatsoever. For finest outcomes, however, do a mix of strength exercises with machines and without machines. For clear distinction, let us talk about weight lifting exercises initially.

Weight lifting is a practical, muscle-building workout as it delivers tension to your muscles via an outer source, the weights. You could additionally quickly gauge your development as the amount of pounds or grams is seen on every weight. As your body strengthens and changes, you could include more weights or substitute your present weights with bigger ones.

To identify how much weight you ought to be lifting, have a go at them initially. The ideal weights for you are those which place tension on your muscles yet do not make you feel too tired.

The ideal exercises for getting faster outcomes when it comes to enhancing metabolism are those which work numerous muscles in your body together. It's not an issue if you wish to concentrate on a specific muscle, however, if you wish to sculpt or tone a particular body part.

There are numerous weight-lifting exercises you could select from to add in your regimen, however, here are several fundamental instances:

1. Bench press-- This is an exercise involving multiple joints, working the major muscles of the chest, triceps and shoulders. To perform this, rest on a bench and have the weight across your chest with your elbows bent at a 90-degree angle. Push the weight up till your arms are straight, then lower it gradually back to your beginning position.

2. Chest fly-- This train the chest, with a focus on external muscles. Rest on a bench with your weights overhead, hands facing inward. Lower the weights down to shoulder level, with your elbows somewhat

bent. Gradually bring the weights up, back to beginning position.

3. Bicep curl-- This is among the most fundamental weight lifting exercises. This places the load on the biceps, as the name recommends. To perform this, hold the weights with your hands facing out. Flex your elbows to bring the weights to your shoulders without touching them. Gradually lower down the weights, however, do not flex the arm completely to maintain a degree of tension.

4. Concentration curl-- This additionally trains the biceps. Kneel on one leg utilizing the leg that is opposite to the hand you are currently training. Hold one weight with one hand and place the other hand on your waist. Put the rear of your working hand's upper arm on the inward thigh of the other leg. You could lean into that leg to elevate your elbow a bit. Lift the weight in front of your shoulder, and after that, gradually lower the arm up until it's practically straight.

5. Overhead press-- This trains the shoulder muscles. Sit or stand straight and hold your weights

with your hands ahead of your eyes and your elbows bent. Bring the weights across your head while making sure your back is straight. Gradually bring the weights down to the beginning stance.

Strength exercises without weights could be integrated with weight lifting exercises for your regimen. Here are certain instances:

1. Squat-- A squat is a compound movement training the quadriceps, gluteus, hamstrings, and the lower back. As a matter of fact, this is among the most reliable strength exercises without weights. From a standing stance, gradually lower your body up until your knees flex at a 90-degree angle. Always keep your feet flat on the floor while performing this. Go back to a standing position gradually too.

2. Pushup-- This is additionally a really reliable and common resistance and strength exercise. While the fundamental one works effectively, including some intricacies can train more muscles. For instance, you may do pushups in between 2 chairs. These train the triceps and chest. Put both feet on a steady

chair, and after that, put both hands on different chairs. The chairs your hands are on could have a 60 centimeter gap. The chair with your feet ought to be lined up with the center of the other 2 chairs. Your body ought to be extended normally from the chair at your feet to the chairs ahead. Gradually bring your chest down-- beyond the surface of the chairs if you are able to!

3. Crunch-- Yes, the standard crunch is an exercise for strength, even though it trains the abs primarily. However, although the crunch is widely recognized, not everybody understands how to do it effectively. To do this properly, rest on a mat, or the floor, with your feet flat on the floor and knees bent. You might place your hands behind your head. Lift your upper body, however, lead with your chest upwards up until you feel your abs contracting. To maintain the tension, do not lift your body up to 90 degrees. Once again, to maintain tension, as you bring down your body, do not allow it to rest on the floor. Rather, maintain yourself a little bit elevated.

For variety, you could additionally attempt exercising with various tools like a medicine ball. In organizing your regimen for strength exercises, refer to the body's muscle groups beneath and identify which you wish to train. Keep in mind, however, that compound movements are still the ideal ways to get quicker metabolism.

1. Biceps-- They are located at the front of your upper arm.

2. Triceps-- They are at the rear of your upper arm.

3.The Pectoralis major-- This is the big, fan-shaped muscle on the front of your upper chest.

4. Deltoids-- These are the caps of your shoulders.

5. Trapezius-- This is on your upper back, often referred to as „traps." The upper trapezius, particularly, goes from the rear of your neck to your shoulder.

6. Rhomboids-- These are muscles in the center of your upper back and situated between the shoulder blades.

7. Lower back-- This consists of the erector spinal column muscles that make it possible for a back extension. This additionally assists in keeping excellent posture.

8. Latisimus dorsi-- These are big muscles which go down your back's middle. When worked out properly, they offer your back an appealing V shape, offering the illusion of a tinier waist.

9. Gluteals-- Additionally referred to as "glutes," the primary muscle here is the gluteus maximus, the muscle on your buttocks.

10. Abdominals-- Naturally! This is where the abdominal fat generally goes, the fat you wish to eliminate permanently. The abs consist of the external obliques, that trace paths down the front and the sides of the abdominal area, and the rectus

abdominus, a flat muscle going over the abdominal area.

11. Hamstrings-- These are on the rear of your thighs.

12. Quadriceps-- These muscles go up the front of your thigh.

13. Hip adductors and abductors -- These lie at your external and inner thigh. Abductors are facing outwards, moving the leg far from your body. Meanwhile, adductors are on the within, pulling the leg to the middle of your body.

14. Calf-- The calf muscles are on the rear of the lower leg. The two calf muscles are the soleus and gastrocnemius. The former offers the calf a round, steady shape as the soleus is a flat muscle beneath the gastrocnemius. After selecting your exercises, you need to consider the intensity level and the length of your exercises. The amount of sets and reps really depend upon your level of tolerance.

Tiredness is an indication that you have actually overtaxed yourself.

Allow yourself to feel the "burn" within your muscles, or the soreness, however, do not force yourself further than you are able to go. Generally, however, the American College of Sports Medicine advises 3 sets or more of strength exercises with 6 to 8 reps for every set for muscle building. If you are a novice, however, it might require time prior to reaching this level. You shouldn't rest more than 45 minutes in between sets for ideal outcomes in boosting metabolism. Your workout regimen could last for just thirty minutes or less while still delivering optimal outcomes.

Now, I wish to highlight that resistance and strength workouts are the healthiest and best methods to build muscles. Do not ever try to find for shortcuts, such as performance-enhancing steroids or drugs with growth hormones. While they might assist in boosting your muscle mass, they could have side effects like liver damage, cardiovascular disease and even untimely death.

It is ideal for you to adhere to the healthy and tested techniques in building muscles.

The advantages of strength workouts are additionally many and not simply restricted to enhancing metabolism. They reduce blood pressure, enhance flexibility and balance, raise your stamina for other things, and decrease your injury risk. As these are exercises for strength, they actually reinforce your bones and muscles!

Interval Training

Yes, these workouts are about "intervals," especially the intervals of rest and high-intensity exercise. In this training, you perform a cardiovascular exercise at the greatest intensity you could handle, then move to mild intensity, do high intensity once again, then mild again, and so forth. Reames refeers to this as "metabolic burst" training, as the abrupt burst you carry out during the high-intensity exercise additionally leads to a calorie-burning burst.

Due to the abrupt "burst" you provide to your body, it additionally unexpectedly discharges energy. The period of rest, on the other hand, is vital for the body to eliminate the waste products in the muscles you are utilizing in the exercise. It is necessary to maintain a mild exercise intensity without resting completely. This is to make sure that the energy release is constant.

Interval training could be performed for practically any kind of cardiovascular exercise-- running, swimming, cycling, and more. For running, period of rest could be brisk walking; for swimming and cycling, the activity could be performed at a slower yet mild pace. The moderate-intensity and high-intensity exercise could additionally be somewhat distinct. For instance, the high-intensity exercise might be going up the stairs briskly while the low-intensity exercise might be going on a flat surface briskly.

Every interval ought to last in between 1 and 4 minutes. The period of rest could be longer or shorter than your high-intensity exercise, based upon your condition. Performing your interval training regimen for thirty minutes overall delivers optimum results. Simply make sure that your moderate-intensity exercise truly still has intensity while enabling your body to recuperate for the following high-intensity bursts. Do your finest during the high-intensity exercise, being nearly breathless is an excellent indication.

A more precise method of figuring out the highest intensity level you could handle is by computing your max heart rate. To get your max heart rate, just deduct your age from 220. Throughout exercise, a heart rate monitor is going to be helpful even though this is optional. To monitor your heart rate by hand, locate your wrist pulse, and then count the beats within 6 seconds. Place zero at the end of the result.

In case you counted 15 beats, your pulse is 150 bpm. Your pulse after high-intensity exercise ought to be 80% of your max heart rate. Your pulse rate throughout mild-intensity exercise ought to constantly be higher than your resting heart rate, or your regular heart rate when you are not exercising.

Once again, to find out your resting heart rate, get your pulse while not exercising. For those who wish to improve metabolism mostly to drop weight, here's the bright side: after a couple of weeks of interval training, you can expect to burn more fat with an exercise of mild intensity.

A study by exercise researcher Jason Talanian stands by this. After 7 interval workouts spread over 2 weeks, subjects boosted their fat-burning by 36 percent via just regular biking exercises. Additionally, based upon Reames, after interval training comes the "metabolic afterburn," and this implies that your body keeps on burning calories for 48 hours following your workout.

Interval training certainly trumps typical cardiovascular training. Additionally, regular cardiovascular exercise typically requires longer as the goal is endurance. Compare this with interval training, which just needs thirty minutes or less and which provides considerable outcomes in simply a couple of weeks.

Putting All of It Together

While you are going to be selecting your particular exercises for the resistance and strength training and interval training, I am going to be advising an exercise schedule and offering you suggestions for your finest application of the exercises.

Beneath would be the ideal weekly regimen:

Day 1: Resistance and strength exercises

Day 2: Interval training

Day 3: Resistance and strength exercises

Day 4: Interval training

Day 5: Resistance and strength exercises

Day 6: Interval training

Day 7: Relax

As you could observe, interval training and strength exercises are performed on alternate days. This is to assist with the restoration of the muscles you utilize. Do not ever, ever perform your strength workout directly after your interval training -- this is going to lessen the procedure of building muscle.

One day without exercise throughout the week is additionally vital for your body to make a complete recovery.

Once again, I wish to stress that you must never ever drive your body to fatigue. Doing so would set off a stress reaction in your body, and that might have major impacts on your metabolism. (The link in between metabolism and stress is going to be talked about in a later part). Additionally, ensure that you breathe properly during the exercises to ensure that your body is calm.

Constantly carry out warm-up exercises prior to your regimen and perform cool-down exercises afterward. For a warm-up, arm circling and moderate cardio would be a fine instance. For a cool-down, a complete body stretch is going to unwind your muscles. Breathing exercises are additionally going to assist in relaxing.

You could add variety to your exercise regimens to work separate muscles and for your own pleasure, specifically if you get burnt out with the identical exercise regimens.

Here are several additional things to consider as you organize your exercise program to ignite your metabolism:

1. Age is not important - Yes, whether you are 20 or 50, you could know the exercise program we went over is going to work for you. For older individuals, your interval training might not be as extreme in the beginning, however, after a bit of time, you simply may be stunned by how far your body is able to go. Taking a look at resistance and strength training, here's something for older individuals to think about: a scientific study carried out at Tufts University reveals that age is not a barrier to muscle building. In their study, 87- to 96-year-old ladies who went through an 8-week strength training course tripled their strength and boosted their muscle mass by 10%.

2. Other exercises are excellent - However, I suggest you use the exercise program talked about here. While it holds true that any physical exertion burns calories, it just has a one-time result. The exercises here, nevertheless, are certain to have a long-lasting impact. Additionally, endurance training is great, however, you are going to get faster and bigger outcomes from interval training.

3. Additional exercise does not imply quicker metabolism. Realistically, additional exercise suggests more calories burned. However, as your objective here is a long-term metabolic boost , you must not be consumed with how much you work out, the quality is what matters. Once again, this deserves repeating-- do not drive yourself beyond your limitations as it is going to push your body into a stress response. Stress has a severe impact on metabolism.

So now you understand the ideal workout program to ignite your metabolism. However, don't stop reading yet-- exercise is just one component of your path to a quicker metabolism.

Metabolism Fuel # 2: Eating Well

Food is your primary energy fuel-- it offers your body the calories it uses to burn or to keep energy. The appropriate food, the appropriate amount, and the appropriate time for consuming are going to offer you the ideal outcomes feasible for your metabolism.

For all those who are attempting to slim down, you have to understand that eating to improve metabolism is significantly distinct from conventional weight-loss diet plans. In conventional diet plans, calories are not your friend, and you need to track your calorie consumption. However, the opposite holds true for the quick metabolism diet.

Calories are now your buddies-- the good calories, at least. Keep in mind the part about exercise? The more muscle you put on, the more calories you burn. And after you have performed interval training for some time, your body additionally burns more calories. So to stay up to date with the calorie-burning, you really need to consume more.

You are going to comprehend this much better later on.

Important Nutrients

Carbs are among the most necessary nutrients for igniting your metabolism. They are the most fundamental fuel for the energy you take in for physical activities. If you work out frequently, carbs are essential. If you are building muscle, carbs are essential. As you advance in your interval training and muscle building, you have to boost your carb consumption. As your body burns more energy, it is going to require more energy from carbs. If the carbs you take in are insufficient, your body is going to switch to muscles for its energy.

Yes, your hard-earned muscles are going to be squandered if you do not take in ample carbs. More than half of your calorie needs ought to originate from carbs.

There are 2 kinds of carbs-- complex and simple. Simple carbs are simpler to absorb and take in compared to complex carbs. If we are to think about the thermic impact of food, which additionally adds to a quicker metabolism, complex carbs are the ones to choose.

And generally, complex carbs are the healthy kind, while simple carbs are normally processed foods filled with sweetening agents and preservatives.

However, simple carbs must not be disregarded totally. Healthy sources of simple carbs are milk, honey and fresh fruit juice. For complex carbs, you have more choices. See the table beneath for certain instances.

COMPLEX CARBOHYDRATES

- Cereal and grains: Oatmeal, whole wheat pasta, whole wheat bread, bran, brown rice, corn.

- Root crops: Potato, taro/yam, sweet potato, manioc

- Vegetables: Broccoli, eggplant, cauliflower, green peppers, cabbage, cucumber, bean sprouts, tomatoes, asparagus, squash, garlic, onion.

Yes, carbs are not all root crops and grains. We have fibrous carbs too-- the veggies. The fiber, though not taken in by the digestive system, assists in the thermic impact. Fiber additionally purifies the body and hence guarantees its smooth performance, consisting of the hormones and enzymes for metabolism.

Protein is one more vital nutrient in the diet for a quicker metabolism. Protein is processed into amino acids, the foundations of cells-- and subsequently, muscles. And, as complex carbs, protein additionally has a thermic impact as it takes a while for the body to break it down.

Beneath are some healthy, outstanding sources of protein:

1. Chicken-- Choose the breast, as it has the greatest quantity of protein. Drumsticks are additionally excellent, though they don't have so much protein. Simply eliminate the skin to do away with cholesterol and saturated fat.

2. Fish-- This is an excellent protein without the bad things, unlike red meat. Apart from having a high protein material, it is additionally great for the heart, especially coldwater fish such as tuna and salmon.

3. Eggs-- Really abundant in protein and inexpensive too. Eggs include all the necessary amino acids for development. Contrary to what some might believe, the high protein material stems mainly from the egg white.

4. Milk-- This is a necessity for anybody who wishes to put on muscle. It is not surprising that toddlers and babies are provided with milk for development. So learn from your youth and enjoy milk.

5. Whey-- It is not a whole food, yet whey has a lot of protein and is additionally healthy. It is a foundation amongst bodybuilders. Whey is offered as powder.

Fats are additionally necessary for quick metabolism. Now, this might raise a couple of eyebrows, particularly amongst those who have actually attempted traditional weight-loss diet plans. This is where the quick metabolism diet plan, once again, sets itself apart. While excessive fat-- particularly unhealthy fat-- is not god, a tiny amount of healthy fats assists hormones in charge of metabolism.

Diet plans that are low in fat result in bad hormone generation, and therefore, slower metabolism.

When including fats to your diet plan, don't forget to have them in their correct location: atop the food pyramid. Healthy fat sources are olive oil, sunflower seeds, avocados, and nuts.

Similar to fats, calcium assists hormones which improve metabolism. Milk, naturally, is the ideal calcium source. Yogurt additionally has a lot of calcium and has other health advantages too.

What to Stay Clear of

Stay clear of empty calories as much as you can. These originated from refined, extremely processed foods-- normally the simple carbs which are not whole natural foods. Empty calories fill you up yet offer no or little nutrients. What's more, these foods typically consist of a great deal of sugar-- and excessive sugar impacts the metabolism considerably.

Simply to drive home the point, beneath are instances of foods with empty calories:

Gums

Pastries

Candies

Biscuits

Chocolate bars

Cakes

Sodas

Junk food

Flavored drinks

White bread, pasta and rice.

Excessive caffeine is additionally bad for your metabolism. It activates a stress reaction. So take it easy with the coffee.

Other Advised Foods

1. Spices-- Red hot pepper and cayenne pepper, particularly, consist of capsaicin, which should boost metabolism up to 25% for 3 hours.

2. Green Tea-- It's not just about anti-oxidants. If drank frequently, green tea could boost the thermic impact of food. Research from the University of Geneva reveals that green tea accelerates fat oxidation along with enhancing metabolism. Green

tea additionally has less caffeine than coffee, whose caffeine level might considerably impact metabolism. For those who don't enjoy the taste, green tea extract is readily offered in pill form.

Water is Key

The old guidance is true for health along with metabolism-- drink at least 8 glasses of water daily.

Dehydration impacts metabolism via a body temperature drop. This drop induces your body to keep fat to assist with preserving or boosting your body temperature.

Additionally, as you are going to be doing more exercise, you require water to maintain your levels of energy. In case you sweat a great deal, you ought to consume more water-- much more than 8 glasses.

Water cleanses the body of contaminants and hence allows body procedures to continue properly, involving metabolism.

Timing is Important

Although you are taking in the appropriate foods, your outcomes are going to be jeopardized if your timing is not ideal. Follow the guidance beneath, and you are going to get the ideal outcomes.

1. Consume a number of meals per day, every 2 and a half hours to 3 hours. To actually take full advantage of the thermic impact of food, you have to consume more than 3 meals. Eating every 3 hours is going to enable the thermic impact to last you during the day, as it takes in between 2 and a half to 3 hours to digest food while protein broken down into amino acids remains in the bloodstream for 3 hours. For the identical number of meals, the magic number for guys is 6 while it is 5 for ladies. Men need 600-900 more calories daily than women.

Do not go over your ideal amount of meals, specifically via late-night snacking. When you are sleeping, your body has a challenging time digesting. Additionally, the calories from your previous meal are kept as fat. Having the final meal light and simpler to digest contrasted to the earlier meals is suggested.

2. Constantly eat breakfast. Your body has actually been in starvation mode throughout your sleep time. To get your metabolism going once again, begin the day properly with a hearty, healthy breakfast. The later you consume your initial meal, the later your metabolism begins.

3. Do not skip meals. Under no conditions can you skip meals, particularly the 3 standard meals. If you have a hectic day and have a difficult time snacking, have "emergency" foods inside your grasp, such as bananas and whole wheat crackers.

Throughout especially busy days, simply a couple of crackers or one banana would be enough as a treat to make sure your metabolism keeps going. A protein shake or fresh fruit shake would additionally suffice.

4. Take one treat or meal after your exercise. A treat or meal with carbs and protein taken within an hour

after your exercise assists with the recuperation of your muscles and the construction of brand-new ones.

5. Do not eat less than 2 and a half hours prior to bedtime. Although metabolism still takes place while sleeping, food digestion is going to be challenging, and your calories are probably going to be kept as fat.

Sample Meal Plans

Beneath are 2 sample meal plans for a day. The key with every meal, especially the primary ones, is to integrate carbs and protein. Portions depend upon your individual everyday calorie needs. Keep in mind, however, that carbs ought to have the largest share in your diet plan-- and these consist of significant portions of veggies!-- followed by protein. Calcium is additionally important. Fats are the final priority. You could have green tea with your meals.

MEAL PLAN 1

8 AM - Meal 1

Poached egg

Oatmeal with banana slivers

11 AM - Meal 2

Protein Shake

3 PM - Meal 3

Skinless chicken breast with olive oil

Steamed broccoli

Potatoes

Brown rice

6 PM - Meal 4

Green beans

9 PM - Meal 5

Sweet potato

Cauliflower

Salmon fillet

MEAL PLAN 2

8 AM - Meal 1

Choice of fruit/s-- blueberry, strawberries and/or banana.

Egg white pancakes (just one or two yolks may be included).

11 AM - Meal 2.

Selection of fruit.

Brown rice.

Yogurt.

3 PM - Meal 3.

Vegetable curry.

6 PM - Meal 4.

Fruit salad with grilled chicken and greens

9 PM - Meal 5.

Chili (made of turkey, salsa and kidney beans).

Steamed vegetables.

Milk (Optional)

These meal plans are here simply to offer you an idea. Produce your own, however, don't forget the principles. You could additionally shift the times here, however, keep in mind not to eat too late during the night.

Beneath are certain things to keep an eye out for in order to have quicker metabolism:

1. Certain foods could just take you so far. Green tea and spicy foods do get some results in increasing metabolism, however, just as an inclusion to a diet plan currently abundant in carbs and protein. Depending on these alone for quicker metabolism is inadequate.

2. Certain foods will not take you there whatsoever. Grapefruit is particularly prominent amongst dieters as its high level of acidity is understood to burn fats. Nevertheless, there is no scientific evidence of this.

3. No supplement is going to increase your metabolism. To those who are taking supplements to increase your metabolism, you might simply be losing your cash. Once again, there is no scientifically shown link in between quicker metabolism and supplements.

4. Diet pills are not an option. For those who wish to drop weight, certain diet pills might burn a bit of fat and manage your cravings. Nevertheless, they do NOT enhance metabolism. Additionally, the disadvantage of diet pills is that when you get

accustomed to a particular dosage, you have to take more to get the identical impact as in the past. A few of those diet plan pills out there might undoubtedly enhance the metabolism, however, they could have severe side effects. Read the container or box thoroughly. Even better, consult your physician. After seeing the unfavorable effects of diet pills, doesn't it seem better enhancing your metabolism in a natural way? You are going to feel and look now on the final part of the program to ignite your metabolism. Keep reading!

Metabolism Fuel # 3: DE-STRESS

You may be questioning what the goal of this part is-- isn't stress meant to be an everyday, common part of life? But that is simply the point. We now reside in a hectic culture driven by due dates and urgency. The more things you get performed in less time, the better. Family, work and leisure have actually ended up being a balancing act. Stress, anxiety, fear and worry are all too typical. Psychological issues like marriage failures, deaths of family members, or struggling relationships are followed by work pressures.

Stress, specifically extended stress exposure, could seriously impact your metabolism, along with your general wellness and health.

Stress and Metabolism

There is a hormone within our body by the name of cortisol, which helps in specific body functions. It helps with the blood pressure regulation, the insulin release for blood sugar stability, a boost of immunity, and appropriate metabolization of glucose. Little boosts of cortisol could be useful, leading to a fast, healthy jolt of immunity and energy, increased memory, and a greater pain threshold. Nevertheless, when excessive cortisol is discharged or if it is discharged frequently, it leads to the following:

Blood sugar imbalances

Greater blood pressure

Reduced immunity

Lower cognitive functionality

Reduction in bone density

A reduction in muscle tissue

Cortisol especially promotes amino acid release from your muscles to be transformed into glucose that is going to work as a source of energy for your body to deal with stress. Your precious muscles are at the grace of cortisol if you don't manage its levels.

The cortisol release is generally activated by stress, whether physical or psychological in nature. Can you recall what we spoke about for your workout regimen? Do not overtax yourself as it sets off the body's stress reaction.

Stress is additionally hazardous to the body as it causes the creation of more acid than the body requires. Our bodies generally have a balance of 20% acid and 80% alkaline. More acid in the body is going to rock that balance.

Excessive acid reduces your immune system and makes you more susceptible to disease. Excessive acid additionally impacts body functions, involving metabolism.

You could successfully manage stress and maintain your cortisol levels healthy and steady, though. When your body enters the stress reaction, it is essential that you assist it in entering into the relaxation reaction.

How to De-Stress

There are lots of methods to de-stress, as there are numerous reasons for stress. Select the ones you like the most:

1. Aromatherapy-- This is especially helpful to allow your stress throughout the day dissipate. Mint and lavender essential oils have outstanding relaxing qualities. A couple of drops combined with water on your oil burner are going to be sufficient. You could additionally mix aromatherapy with meditation. As the scent covers you, feel it gradually absorbing your fatigue and concerns.

As the scent leaves later on, picture your concerns and exhaustion additionally disappearing with it.

You could additionally quickly unwind with aromatherapy throughout work. Place a couple of drops on some tissue paper and breathe in. Shut your eyes while doing this.

2. Massage-- This is additionally appropriately called touch therapy. A massage is additionally advantageous as it loosens up the joints and muscles which might have tightened because of constant stress. Back muscles are especially prone to this.

You can additionally mix aromatherapy and massage -- you could ask the masseuse or masseur to utilize essential oils for your massage. Peppermint is especially outstanding. Aside from its scent, it has a chilling impact on the body when utilized as a massage oil.

3. Music therapy-- Place some mild, peaceful music on your player, lie or sit in a comfy position, shut your eyes, and allow the music to wash over you. Picture it removing your worries, concerns and anxieties. An excellent alternative to calming music are the natural sounds, such as ocean waves. If you

discover that you delight in relaxing on the beach, then bring the beach home with you by means of recordings of waves.

4. Imagery-- Picture that you are a kite gradually drifting and ascending through the air. You drift in the bright blue sky in harmony and balance. After a bit of time, feel yourself gradually sliding downwards, and after that, gently touching the ground. The above imagery is especially useful not just for relaxing yet for replicating an excellent stress response -- notice that the movement of the kite is in harmony with the wind, although the identical wind could additionally make the kite spin out of control.

Another imagery method is to envision a gorgeous natural scene such as a mountaintop, a remote island, or a tropical rainforest. Envision yourself, from a first-person viewpoint, going through the location and absorbing all the appeal. You can change the location you go to each time you utilize this strategy, or you could choose one and make it your sanctuary-- the location you run to throughout stressful moments. For the long run:

1. Think positive!-- Thoughts considerably affect your health and wellness. Your thoughts could really manifest into truth, as claimed by modern speakers, philosophers and even researchers. Bad thoughts could manifest adversely, while positive thoughts can manifest favorably. So if you will think, why not think about enjoyable things?

In case you have anxieties regarding something, such as an approaching presentation for work, picture yourself-- from the first-person point of view-- providing an outstanding, perfect presentation. Picture the responses of your audience. Feel the sensations as if you were there already. Images are more effective than words.

2. Release negative feelings. Wallowing in negative feelings equates to additional acid in the body. It's no surprise that fear and tension result in indigestion or heartburn, while chronic worry and/or animosity makes you more vulnerable to hypertension.

Nevertheless, do not subdue your feelings, although some might appear illogical to you. Doing so additionally results in greater levels of acid. Feel the sensation, express it via healthy catharsis in a secure environment if you feel the requirement (e.g., yelling into a pillow)-- and let it go. Yes, the secret here is to let go.

3. Meditate every day-- Turn meditation into a routine. In the long run, meditation brings you comfort and makes you more capable to deal with stress. It doesn't have to be an intricate meditation-- emptiness of mind and stillness is the secret. Sit in a comfy position and breathe gradually, deeply. Concentrate on every part of your body and feel it discharge its tension. After you feel adequately unwinded, you could quietly chant a simple word without any specific psychological attachment for you-- for instance, "tree.".

Or, you could, in fact, say a letter, such as B. Repeat this letter or word in your head for approximately one minute. Then sit and allow thoughts to come to your head. See your thoughts as if you were separated from them, as if they were another individual's thoughts. This is to ensure that you do not stay on a thought. Simply naturally, objectively, permit any thought to get in and leave your head. In case you get to a state of emptiness, where you don't think about anything, good job! It might take a while for you to get to this point, however.

4. Take up yoga. Not just is this an outstanding stress-buster, it additionally ignites your metabolism. Thyroid and the endocryne system assist with managing metabolism. Yoga has numerous positions which offer a healthy twist and compression to your endocrine organs, thus reinforcing them for metabolism.

For relaxation from stress, however, a great yoga position is the corpse position. As its name advises, you ought to lie as a corpse. Unleash all tension from your body. The corpse position is, in fact, an excellent way to end your yoga regimen.

5. Plan ahead-- In case the reason for your stress is repeating, plan ahead. After you have actually determined the reason for your tension, ask yourself if there is any method to stay away from it. For instance, one reason for your stress might be the early morning rush-hour traffic. To be at peace as you are getting to work, you need to leave early.

Then you remember you watch tv each night, often late into the night. To stay clear of tension in the early morning, you conclude that you could reduce your tv time and hit the hay earlier the night prior.

Also, in case your body goes through stress because of something like long working hours, you ought to customize your diet plan while still knowing the principles of the quick metabolism diet. You specifically want Vitamin C, as this assists the body in coping throughout stress. Load up on strawberries and citrus fruits.

For veggies, sweet red pepper is an exceptional Vitamin C source. Aside from that, your diet plan stays identical-- load up on complex carbs, especially fibrous ones, and consume protein.

Sleep is Essential

Sleep is the time your body totally recuperates from your day. This is additionally the time when your muscles develop-- yes, they do not develop throughout your workout, but while you remain in bed. Without a lot of sleep, your muscles grow really little even if you place in a lot of effort when working out.

Shortage of sleep is going to additionally stop your body from remaining in top shape and is going to impact your energy for working out additionally. You may find yourself burning out quickly, even after a couple of reps or sets.

Additionally, scientific studies reveal that the shortage of sleep impacts carbohydrate metabolization. Glucose is not metabolized as much, leading to increased appetite and reduced total metabolism.

It is necessary for you to get at least 8 hours of sleep each night for the body to completely re-energize for the following day. Even though individuals' circadian rhythms might vary, the typical circadian rhythm is from 10 pm to 6 am. This is the ideal time for muscles to develop. So sleep early to boost your metabolic process!

For some, de-stressing might be the hardest portion of the program to enhance metabolism. What if stress has ended up being so much a part of your everyday life that making major modifications in your way of life is hard? You can take things gradually. The least you have to do, however, is to discover a bit of silent time to yourself each day. It could be as little as 10 minutes. Utilize those 10 minutes simply to practice meditation and unwind.

Meditation goes far. Even 10 minutes daily assists you to cope much better with stress. Studies reveal that individuals who practice meditation frequently are less stressed out and are more able to meet life's requirements.

Don't allow your sleep "debt" build up. Sleep "debt" results in bad cognitive function and bad health in general. Your body procedures don't function as effectively as they ought to-- which involves metabolism. Take some time to de-stress. It increases your metabolism while it also enhances your general health.

So now you understand the whole program. However, we are not done just yet!

Conclusion

You have actually discovered all you have to do - now is the ideal time to begin.

To conclude, you have actually discovered that metabolism is the procedure of transforming calories into energy for storage or instant utilization. You now understand that metabolism is an important function, working each second -- even when you are asleep. And you now understand the general metabolism equation-- physical activity + basal metabolism + the thermic impact of food, along with what elements affect your metabolic rate.

Now you currently have the understanding of how to enhance your metabolic process:

Exercise Intelligently

- Build muscle with a mix of resistance and strength workouts with weights and without any weights. Utilize exercises which train the most muscle groups at once. (2-3 sets, with 6-8 repetitions each).

- Boost calorie-burning via cardiovascular exercise and interval training. Alternate with mild-intensity and high-intensity exercise. (thirty minutes, with one to four minutes per interval).

- Do the two exercises on alternate days over the course of the week. Set aside a single day for complete rest without exercise.

Eat Well.

- Stock up on protein and carbs, since these are the drivers of metabolism.

- Incorporate healthy fats and calcium into your eating plan.

- Timing is necessary.

  - Constantly eat breakfast to get your metabolism started.
  - Consume 5 to 6 meals in a day, every 2 and a half to 3 hours. Never ever skip meals.
  - Drink at least 8 glasses of water daily.
  - Take one meal or treat inside an hour after your daily workout.

De-stress.

- Re-charge via "sensation therapy" (aromatherapy, music and massage) and imagery.

- For long-lasting enhancement, practice meditation every day, start yoga and think positively. Do not dwell on unfavorable feelings. Plan ahead to stay away from nerve-racking scenarios.

So there it is. What you now have to do is "excuse-proof" metabolic program to guarantee that you get the ideal outcomes. In times when you don't feel much inspiration, return to the scene which I asked you to envision, yourself after finishing the program. Though people's bodies are different, you are going to probably notice the outcomes in 3 or 4 weeks-- and perhaps even 2 weeks.

Best of luck!

I hope that you enjoyed reading through this book and that you have found it useful. If you want to share your thoughts on this book, you can do so by leaving a review on the Amazon page. Have a great rest of the day.

Printed in Great Britain
by Amazon